Bef

Starting Weight:

Starting BMI: Ending BMI:

Measurements

Neck: Neck:

Bust: Bust:

Hips: Hips:

Waist: Waist:

Thigh: Thigh:

Arm: Arm:

Note To Future Self

I want and deserve this because:

Month Goals

Starting Weight: Starting BMI:

4 WK WEIGHT LOSS GOAL:_____

Non Scale Goal:

Exercise Goal:

Action Plan:

Reward:

30 Day Habit Tracker

Habits To Grow: Habits To Cut:

Habit:

1   2   3   4   5   6   7   8   9   10   11   12   13   14   15   16   17
18   19   20   21   22   23   24   25   26   27   28   29   30

Habit:

1   2   3   4   5   6   7   8   9   10   11   12   13   14   15   16   17
18   19   20   21   22   23   24   25   26   27   28   29   30

Habit:

1   2   3   4   5   6   7   8   9   10   11   12   13   14   15   16   17
18   19   20   21   22   23   24   25   26   27   28   29   30

Habit:

1   2   3   4   5   6   7   8   9   10   11   12   13   14   15   16   17
18   19   20   21   22   23   24   25   26   27   28   29   30

MONTH:

WEEK AT A GLANCE

WEIGHT: _____

EVENTS TO PLAN AROUND	MINI GOAL THIS WEEK
☐	
☐	
☐	**WORDS OF SELF ENCOURAGEMENT**
☐	
☐	

WEEK MEAL PLAN

	BKFST.	LUNCH	DINNER	SNACKS	CALS.
MON.					
TUE.					
WED.					
THUR.					

	BKFST.	LUNCH	DINNER	SNACKS	CALS.
FRI.					
SAT.					
SUN.					

SELF LOVE PROMPT:

NO SELF-CRITICISM THIS WEEK! INSTEAD STAND IN FRONT OF THE MIRROR AS OFTEN AS POSSIBLE THIS WEEK AND REMIND YOURSELF THAT YOU'RE AMAZING. SAY "I LOVE YOU", "YOUR ARE BEAUTIFUL" OR ANY OTHER AFFIRMATIONS YOU WOULD LIKE AND KEEP REPEATING IT BECAUSE IT'S SO EASY TO FORGET.

Grocery List

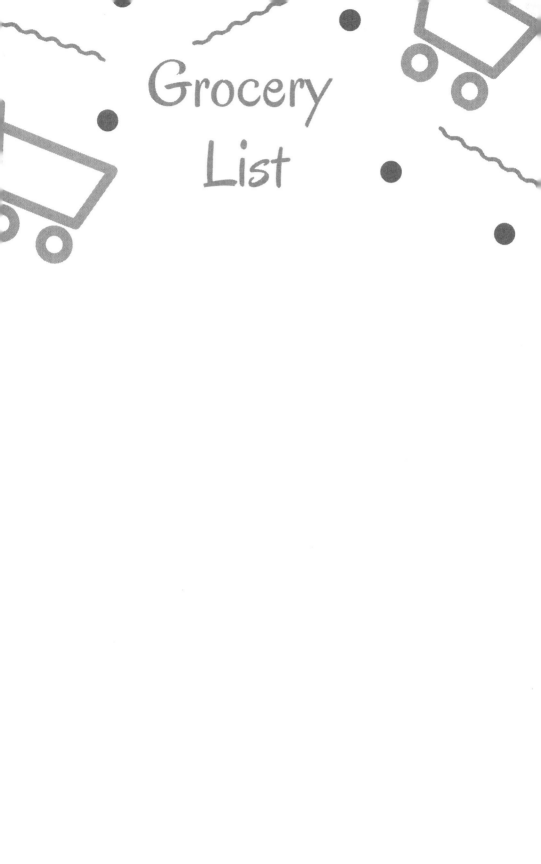

DATE:

YESTERDAY'S WIN:

TODAY'S GOAL:

1 THING I'M GRATEFUL FOR:

TO DO'S:

EXERCISE:

BREAKFAST

LUNCH

DINNER

SNACKS

WATER

DATE:

YESTERDAY'S WIN:

TODAY'S GOAL:

I THING I'M GRATEFUL FOR:

TO DO'S:

EXERCISE:

BREAKFAST

LUNCH

DINNER

SNACKS

WATER

DATE:

YESTERDAY'S WIN:

TODAY'S GOAL:

1 THING I'M GRATEFUL FOR:

TO DO'S:

EXERCISE:

BREAKFAST

LUNCH

DINNER

SNACKS

WATER

DATE:

YESTERDAY'S WIN:

TODAY'S GOAL:

I THING I'M GRATEFUL FOR:

TO DO'S:

EXERCISE:

BREAKFAST

LUNCH

DINNER

SNACKS

WATER

DATE:

YESTERDAY'S WIN:

TODAY'S GOAL:

I THING I'M GRATEFUL FOR:

TO DO'S:

EXERCISE:

BREAKFAST

LUNCH

DINNER

SNACKS

WATER

DATE:

YESTERDAY'S WIN:

TODAY'S GOAL:

I THING I'M GRATEFUL FOR:

TO DO'S:

EXERCISE:

BREAKFAST

LUNCH

DINNER

SNACKS

WATER

DATE:

YESTERDAY'S WIN:

TODAY'S GOAL:

I THING I'M GRATEFUL FOR:

TO DO'S:

EXERCISE:

BREAKFAST

LUNCH

DINNER

SNACKS

WATER

Weekly Reflection

3 Wins This Week:

What Needs Improvement?

Actions Towards Improvement:

WEEK AT A GLANCE

WEIGHT: _____

EVENTS TO PLAN AROUND	MINI GOAL THIS WEEK
☐	
☐	
☐	**WORDS OF SELF ENCOURAGEMENT**
☐	
☐	

WEEK MEAL PLAN

	BKFST.	LUNCH	DINNER	SNACKS	CALS.
MON.					
TUE.					
WED.					
THUR.					

	BKFST.	LUNCH	DINNER	SNACKS	CALS.
FRI.					
SAT.					
SUN.					

SELF LOVE PROMPT:

CLUTTER CAN MAKE YOU LESS PRODUCTIVE DURING THE
DAY WHILE ALSO CAUSING EXTRA STRESS. AS YOU GO
THROUGH YOUR WEEK SHOW SOME SELF LOVE BY
REDUCING THE CLUTTER. GET RID OF ANYTHING YOU
DON'T NEED OR NO LONGER WANT.

Grocery List

DATE:

YESTERDAY'S WIN:

BREAKFAST

TODAY'S GOAL:

I THING I'M GRATEFUL FOR:

LUNCH

TO DO'S:

DINNER

EXERCISE:

SNACKS

WATER

DATE:

YESTERDAY'S WIN:

TODAY'S GOAL:

I THING I'M GRATEFUL FOR:

TO DO'S:

EXERCISE:

BREAKFAST

LUNCH

DINNER

SNACKS

WATER

DATE:

YESTERDAY'S WIN:

TODAY'S GOAL:

1 THING I'M GRATEFUL FOR:

TO DO'S:

EXERCISE:

BREAKFAST

LUNCH

DINNER

SNACKS

WATER

DATE:

YESTERDAY'S WIN:

TODAY'S GOAL:

I THING I'M GRATEFUL FOR:

TO DO'S:

EXERCISE:

BREAKFAST

LUNCH

DINNER

SNACKS

WATER

DATE:

YESTERDAY'S WIN:

TODAY'S GOAL:

I THING I'M GRATEFUL FOR:

TO DO'S:

EXERCISE:

BREAKFAST

LUNCH

DINNER

SNACKS

WATER

DATE:

YESTERDAY'S WIN:

TODAY'S GOAL:

I THING I'M GRATEFUL FOR:

TO DO'S:

EXERCISE:

BREAKFAST

LUNCH

DINNER

SNACKS

WATER

DATE:

YESTERDAY'S WIN:

BREAKFAST

TODAY'S GOAL:

I THING I'M GRATEFUL FOR:

LUNCH

TO DO'S:

DINNER

EXERCISE:

SNACKS

WATER

Weekly Reflection

3 Wins This Week:

What Needs Improvement?

Actions Towards Improvement:

WEEK AT A GLANCE

WEIGHT: _____

EVENTS TO PLAN AROUND	MINI GOAL THIS WEEK
☐	
☐	
☐	**WORDS OF SELF ENCOURAGEMENT**
☐	
☐	

WEEK MEAL PLAN

	BKFST.	LUNCH	DINNER	SNACKS	CALS.
MON.					
TUE.					
WED.					
THUR.					

	BKFST.	LUNCH	DINNER	SNACKS	CALS.
FRI.					
SAT.					
SUN.					

SELF LOVE PROMPT:

SCHEDULE SOME TIME TO BE WITH NATURE THIS WEEK.
GO FOR A WALK IN A PARK, GET TO A BODY OF WATER OR
SPEND SOME TIME ON YOUR PORCH. JUST DO SOMETHING
THAT GETS YOU OUTSIDE. TAKE YOUR SHOES OFF AND
ENJOY THE FEELING OF THE EARTH BENEATH YOU
HOLDING YOUR WEIGHT.

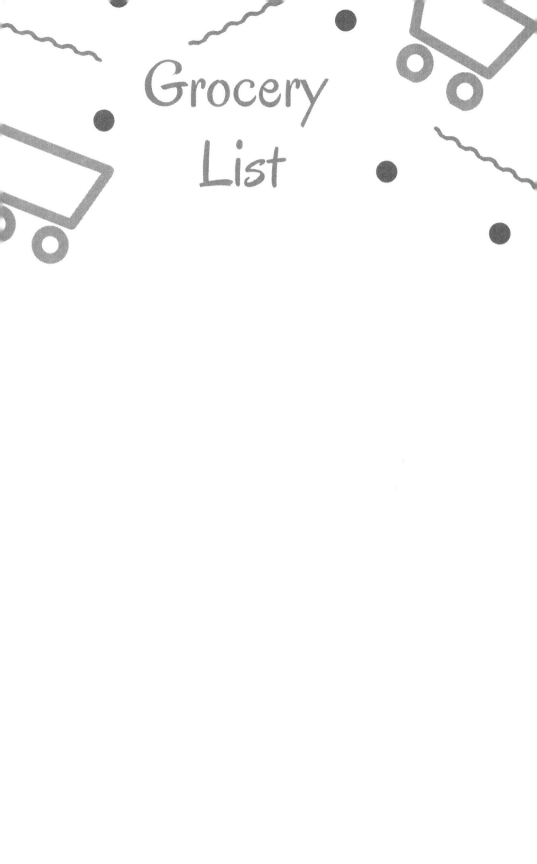

Grocery List

DATE:

YESTERDAY'S WIN:

TODAY'S GOAL:

I THING I'M GRATEFUL FOR:

TO DO'S:

EXERCISE:

BREAKFAST

LUNCH

DINNER

SNACKS

WATER

DATE:

YESTERDAY'S WIN:

TODAY'S GOAL:

I THING I'M GRATEFUL FOR:

TO DO'S:

EXERCISE:

BREAKFAST

LUNCH

DINNER

SNACKS

WATER

DATE:

YESTERDAY'S WIN:

BREAKFAST

TODAY'S GOAL:

I THING I'M GRATEFUL FOR:

LUNCH

TO DO'S:

DINNER

EXERCISE:

SNACKS

WATER

DATE:

YESTERDAY'S WIN:

TODAY'S GOAL:

I THING I'M GRATEFUL FOR:

TO DO'S:

EXERCISE:

BREAKFAST

LUNCH

DINNER

SNACKS

WATER

DATE:

YESTERDAY'S WIN:

TODAY'S GOAL:

I THING I'M GRATEFUL FOR:

TO DO'S:

EXERCISE:

BREAKFAST

LUNCH

DINNER

SNACKS

WATER

DATE:

YESTERDAY'S WIN:

TODAY'S GOAL:

I THING I'M GRATEFUL FOR:

TO DO'S:

EXERCISE:

BREAKFAST

LUNCH

DINNER

SNACKS

WATER

DATE:

YESTERDAY'S WIN:

BREAKFAST

TODAY'S GOAL:

I THING I'M GRATEFUL FOR:

LUNCH

TO DO'S:

DINNER

EXERCISE:

SNACKS

WATER

Weekly Reflection

3 Wins This Week:

What Needs Improvement?

Actions Towards Improvement:

WEEK AT A GLANCE

WEIGHT: _____

EVENTS TO PLAN AROUND

MINI GOAL THIS WEEK

WORDS OF SELF ENCOURAGEMENT

WEEK MEAL PLAN

	BKFST.	LUNCH	DINNER	SNACKS	CALS.
MON.					
TUE.					
WED.					
THUR.					

	BKFST.	LUNCH	DINNER	SNACKS	CALS.
FRI.					
SAT.					
SUN.					

SELF LOVE PROMPT:

AS YOU GO THROUGH YOUR WEEK NOTICE THE PEOPLE
AND PLACES THAT YOU FEEL DRAIN YOU. CHECK IN WITH
YOUR MIND BEFORE EXPOSING YOURSELF TO THESE
SITUATIONS. CREATING BOUNDARIES CAN BE THE
BIGGEST STEP TO SELF-LOVE. START CREATING NEW
BOUNDARIES THAT ARE NEEDED IN YOUR LIFE.

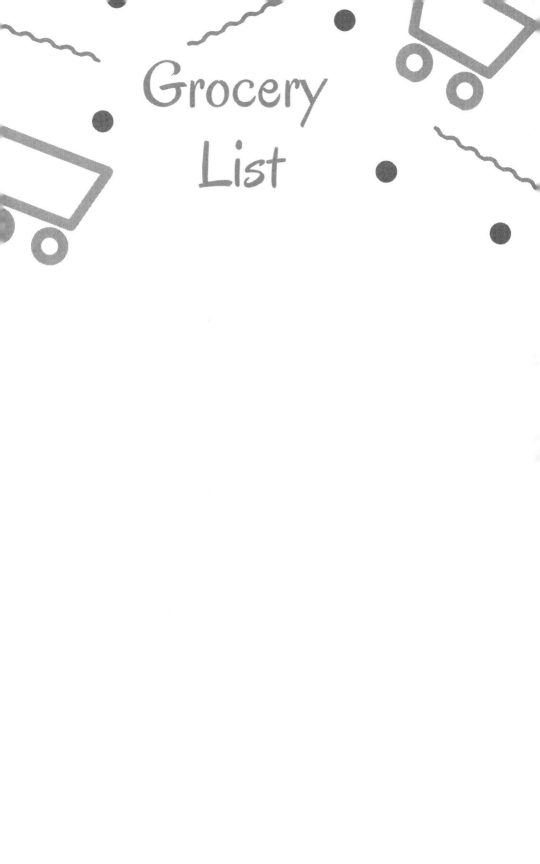

Grocery List

DATE:

YESTERDAY'S WIN:

TODAY'S GOAL:

I THING I'M GRATEFUL FOR:

TO DO'S:

EXERCISE:

BREAKFAST

LUNCH

DINNER

SNACKS

WATER

DATE:

YESTERDAY'S WIN:

TODAY'S GOAL:

1 THING I'M GRATEFUL FOR:

TO DO'S:

EXERCISE:

BREAKFAST

LUNCH

DINNER

SNACKS

WATER

DATE:

YESTERDAY'S WIN:

TODAY'S GOAL:

I THING I'M GRATEFUL FOR:

TO DO'S:

EXERCISE:

BREAKFAST

LUNCH

DINNER

SNACKS

WATER

DATE:

YESTERDAY'S WIN:

TODAY'S GOAL:

I THING I'M GRATEFUL FOR:

TO DO'S:

EXERCISE:

BREAKFAST

LUNCH

DINNER

SNACKS

WATER

DATE:

YESTERDAY'S WIN:

TODAYS GOAL:

I THING I'M GRATEFUL FOR:

TO DO'S:

EXERCISE:

BREAKFAST

LUNCH

DINNER

SNACKS

WATER

DATE:

YESTERDAY'S WIN:

TODAY'S GOAL:

I THING I'M GRATEFUL FOR:

TO DO'S:

EXERCISE:

BREAKFAST

LUNCH

DINNER

SNACKS

WATER

DATE:

YESTERDAY'S WIN:

TODAY'S GOAL:

I THING I'M GRATEFUL FOR:

TO DO'S:

EXERCISE:

BREAKFAST

LUNCH

DINNER

SNACKS

WATER

Weekly Reflection

3 Wins This Week:

What Needs Improvement?

Actions Towards Improvement:

End Of Month Check In

Ending Weight: Ending BMI:

Non Scale Victories This Month :

Updated Measurements

Neck: Waist:

Bust: Thigh:

Hips: Arm:

How Do You Feel?

Month Goals

Starting Weight: Starting BMI:

4 WK WEIGHT LOSS GOAL:_____

Non Scale Goal:

Exercise Goal:

Action Plan:

Reward:

30 Day Habit Tracker

Habits To Grow: Habits To Cut:

Habit:

1 2 3 4 5 6 7 8 9 10 11 12 13 14 15 16 17
18 19 20 21 22 23 24 25 26 27 28 29 30

Habit:

1 2 3 4 5 6 7 8 9 10 11 12 13 14 15 16 17
18 19 20 21 22 23 24 25 26 27 28 29 30

Habit:

1 2 3 4 5 6 7 8 9 10 11 12 13 14 15 16 17
18 19 20 21 22 23 24 25 26 27 28 29 30

Habit:

1 2 3 4 5 6 7 8 9 10 11 12 13 14 15 16 17
18 19 20 21 22 23 24 25 26 27 28 29 30

NOTES

MONTH:

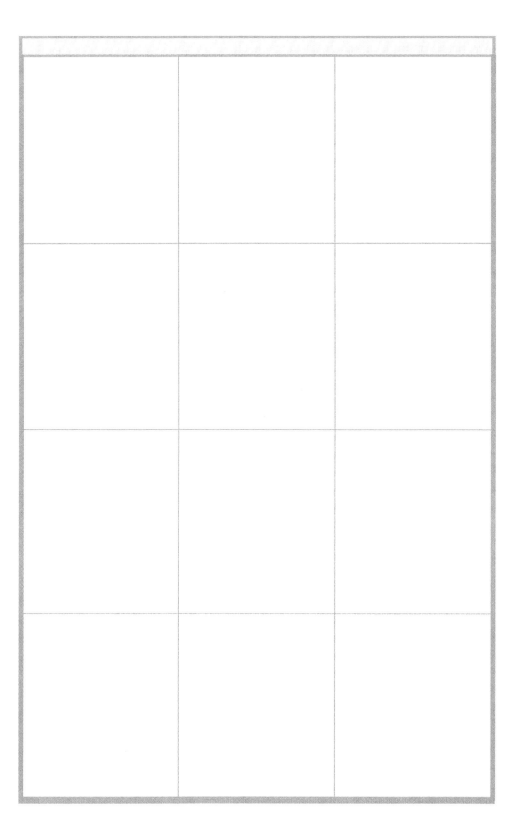

WEEK AT A GLANCE

WEIGHT: _____

EVENTS TO PLAN AROUND

- [ ]
- [ ]
- [ ]
- [ ]
- [ ]

MINI GOAL THIS WEEK

WORDS OF SELF ENCOURAGEMENT

WEEK MEAL PLAN

	BKFST.	LUNCH	DINNER	SNACKS	CALS.
MON.					
TUE.					
WED.					
THUR.					

	BKFST.	LUNCH	DINNER	SNACKS	CALS.
FRI.					
SAT.					
SUN.					

SELF LOVE PROMPT:

FIND I HOUR EACH DAY TO DISCONNECT. THIS CAN BE IN
THE MORNINGS, YOUR LUNCH BREAK OR AN HOUR BEFORE
BED. TURN YOUR PHONE AND OTHER ELECTRONICS OFF.
SPEND TIME SITTING STILL, READING A BOOK OR
ENJOYING THE COMPANY OF A LOVED ONE.

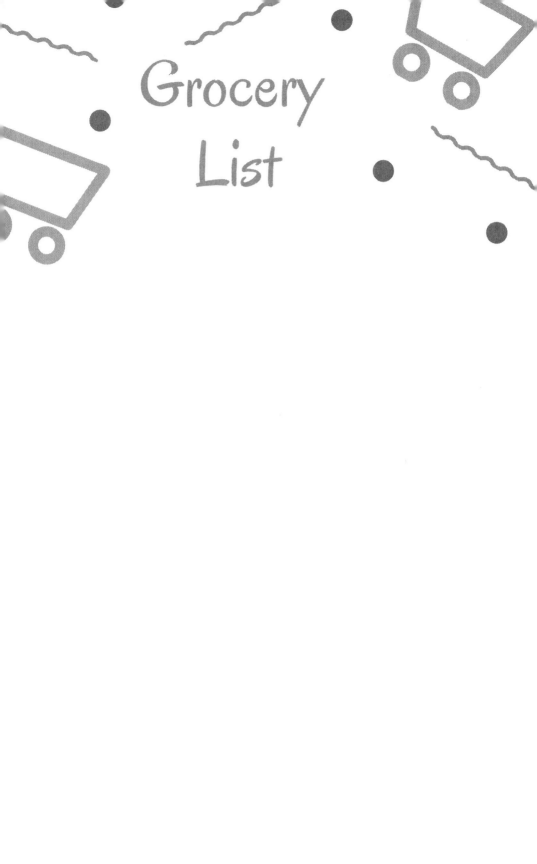

Grocery
List

DATE:

YESTERDAY'S WIN:

TODAY'S GOAL:

1 THING I'M GRATEFUL FOR:

TO DO'S:

EXERCISE:

BREAKFAST

LUNCH

DINNER

SNACKS

WATER

DATE:

YESTERDAY'S WIN:

TODAY'S GOAL:

I THING I'M GRATEFUL FOR:

TO DO'S:

EXERCISE:

BREAKFAST

LUNCH

DINNER

SNACKS

WATER

DATE:

YESTERDAY'S WIN:

TODAY'S GOAL:

I THING I'M GRATEFUL FOR:

TO DO'S:

EXERCISE:

BREAKFAST

LUNCH

DINNER

SNACKS

WATER

DATE:

YESTERDAY'S WIN:

TODAY'S GOAL:

I THING I'M GRATEFUL FOR:

TO DO'S:

EXERCISE:

BREAKFAST

LUNCH

DINNER

SNACKS

WATER

DATE:

YESTERDAY'S WIN:

TODAY'S GOAL:

I THING I'M GRATEFUL FOR:

TO DO'S:

EXERCISE:

BREAKFAST

LUNCH

DINNER

SNACKS

WATER

DATE:

YESTERDAY'S WIN:

TODAY'S GOAL:

I THING I'M GRATEFUL FOR:

TO DO'S:

EXERCISE:

BREAKFAST

LUNCH

DINNER

SNACKS

WATER

DATE:

YESTERDAY'S WIN:

TODAY'S GOAL:

I THING I'M GRATEFUL FOR:

TO DO'S:

EXERCISE:

BREAKFAST

LUNCH

DINNER

SNACKS

WATER

Weekly Reflection

3 Wins This Week:

What Needs Improvement?

Actions Towards Improvement:

WEEK AT A GLANCE

WEIGHT: _____

EVENTS TO PLAN AROUND	MINI GOAL THIS WEEK
☐	
☐	
☐	**WORDS OF SELF ENCOURAGEMENT**
☐	
☐	

WEEK MEAL PLAN

	BKFST.	LUNCH	DINNER	SNACKS	CALS.
MON.					
TUE.					
WED.					
THUR.					

	BKFST.	LUNCH	DINNER	SNACKS	CALS.
FRI.					
SAT.					
SUN.					

SELF LOVE PROMPT:

MONDAY MORNING WRITE YOUR FAVORITE AFFIRMATIONS
ON STICKY NOTES. PUT THEM WHERE YOU'LL SEE THEM
EVERY DAY. YOUR BATHROOM MIRROR OR FRIDGE ARE
GREAT PLACES TO STICK THEM! SEEING THESE
THROUGHOUT THE WEEK WILL BE A GREAT BOOST.

Grocery List

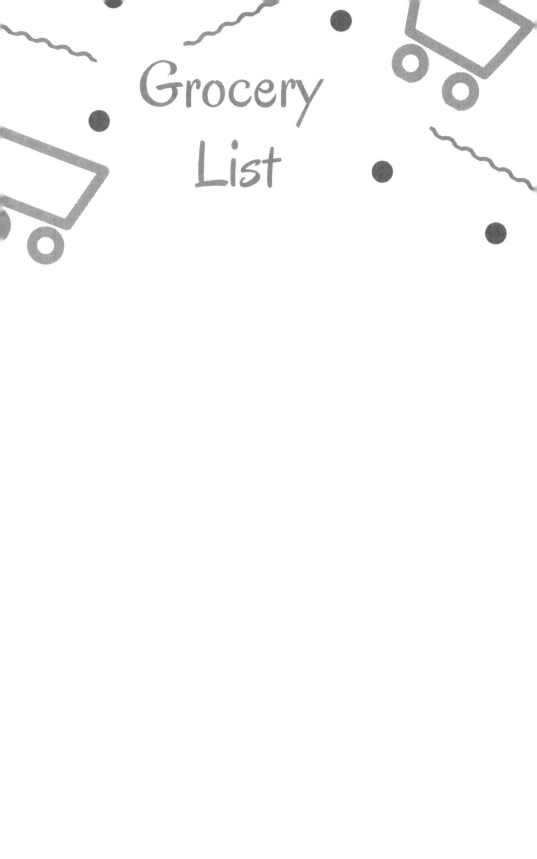

DATE:

YESTERDAY'S WIN:

TODAY'S GOAL:

I THING I'M GRATEFUL FOR:

TO DO'S:

EXERCISE:

BREAKFAST

LUNCH

DINNER

SNACKS

WATER

DATE:

YESTERDAY'S WIN:

TODAY'S GOAL:

I THING I'M GRATEFUL FOR:

TO DO'S:

EXERCISE:

BREAKFAST

LUNCH

DINNER

SNACKS

WATER

DATE:

YESTERDAY'S WIN:

TODAY'S GOAL:

I THING I'M GRATEFUL FOR:

TO DO'S:

EXERCISE:

BREAKFAST

LUNCH

DINNER

SNACKS

WATER

DATE:

YESTERDAY'S WIN:

TODAY'S GOAL:

I THING I'M GRATEFUL FOR:

TO DO'S:

EXERCISE:

BREAKFAST

LUNCH

DINNER

SNACKS

WATER

DATE:

YESTERDAY'S WIN:

BREAKFAST

TODAY'S GOAL:

LUNCH

I THING I'M GRATEFUL FOR:

TO DO'S:

DINNER

EXERCISE:

SNACKS

WATER

DATE:

YESTERDAY'S WIN:

TODAY'S GOAL:

I THING I'M GRATEFUL FOR:

TO DO'S:

EXERCISE:

BREAKFAST

LUNCH

DINNER

SNACKS

WATER

DATE:

YESTERDAY'S WIN:

TODAY'S GOAL:

I THING I'M GRATEFUL FOR:

TO DO'S:

EXERCISE:

BREAKFAST

LUNCH

DINNER

SNACKS

WATER

Weekly Reflection

3 Wins This Week:

What Needs Improvement?

Actions Towards Improvement:

WEEK AT A GLANCE

WEIGHT: _____

EVENTS TO PLAN AROUND	MINI GOAL THIS WEEK
☐	
☐	
☐	**WORDS OF SELF ENCOURAGEMENT**
☐	
☐	

WEEK MEAL PLAN

	BKFST.	LUNCH	DINNER	SNACKS	CALS.
MON.					
TUE.					
WED.					
THUR.					

	BKFST.	LUNCH	DINNER	SNACKS	CALS.
FRI.					
SAT.					
SUN.					

SELF LOVE PROMPT:

FIND SOME TIME TO WRITE A THANK YOU LETTER TO YOUR
BODY FOR ALL IT IS CAPABLE OF! THIS WILL ALLOW YOU
TO THINK KINDLY AND GENTLY TOWARDS YOUR BODY.
PUSH NEGATIVE THOUGHTS OUT OF YOUR HEAD IF THEY
COME UP. ONLY FOCUS ON THE POSITIVE AND WHAT YOU
ARE THANKFUL FOR.

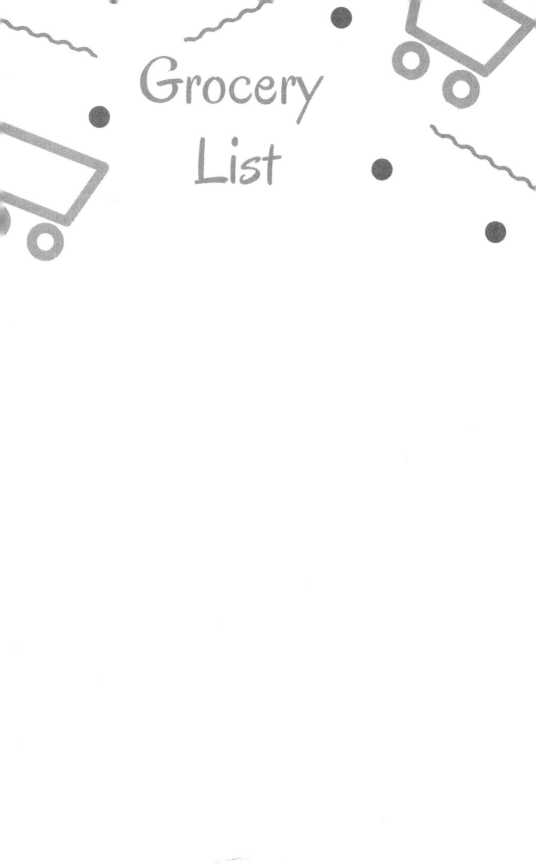

Grocery List

DATE:

YESTERDAY'S WIN:

TODAY'S GOAL:

I THING I'M GRATEFUL FOR:

TO DO'S:

EXERCISE:

BREAKFAST

LUNCH

DINNER

SNACKS

WATER

DATE:

YESTERDAY'S WIN:

TODAY'S GOAL:

I THING I'M GRATEFUL FOR:

TO DO'S:

EXERCISE:

BREAKFAST

LUNCH

DINNER

SNACKS

WATER

DATE:

YESTERDAY'S WIN:

TODAY'S GOAL:

I THING I'M GRATEFUL FOR:

TO DO'S:

EXERCISE:

BREAKFAST

LUNCH

DINNER

SNACKS

WATER

DATE:

YESTERDAY'S WIN:

TODAY'S GOAL:

I THING I'M GRATEFUL FOR:

TO DO'S:

EXERCISE:

BREAKFAST

LUNCH

DINNER

SNACKS

WATER

DATE:

YESTERDAY'S WIN:

TODAY'S GOAL:

I THING I'M GRATEFUL FOR:

TO DO'S:

EXERCISE:

BREAKFAST

LUNCH

DINNER

SNACKS

WATER

DATE:

YESTERDAY'S WIN:

BREAKFAST

TODAY'S GOAL:

I THING I'M GRATEFUL FOR:

LUNCH

TO DO'S:

DINNER

EXERCISE:

SNACKS

WATER

DATE:

YESTERDAY'S WIN:

TODAY'S GOAL:

I THING I'M GRATEFUL FOR:

TO DO'S:

EXERCISE:

BREAKFAST

LUNCH

DINNER

SNACKS

WATER

Weekly Reflection

3 Wins This Week:

What Needs Improvement?

Actions Towards Improvement:

WEEK AT A GLANCE

WEIGHT: _____

EVENTS TO PLAN AROUND	MINI GOAL THIS WEEK
☐	
☐	
☐	**WORDS OF SELF ENCOURAGEMENT**
☐	
☐	

WEEK MEAL PLAN

	BKFST.	LUNCH	DINNER	SNACKS	CALS.
MON.					
TUE.					
WED.					
THUR.					

	BKFST.	LUNCH	DINNER	SNACKS	CALS.
FRI.					
SAT.					
SUN.					

SELF LOVE PROMPT:

FIND A NIGHT THIS WEEK TO FOCUS ON YOURSELF. GET
OUT YOUR FAVORITE NATURAL FACE MASK, PAINT YOUR
NAILS, AND DO SOMETHING THAT MAKES YOU FEEL
PAMPERED. SCHEDULE IN SOME YOU TIME.

Grocery List

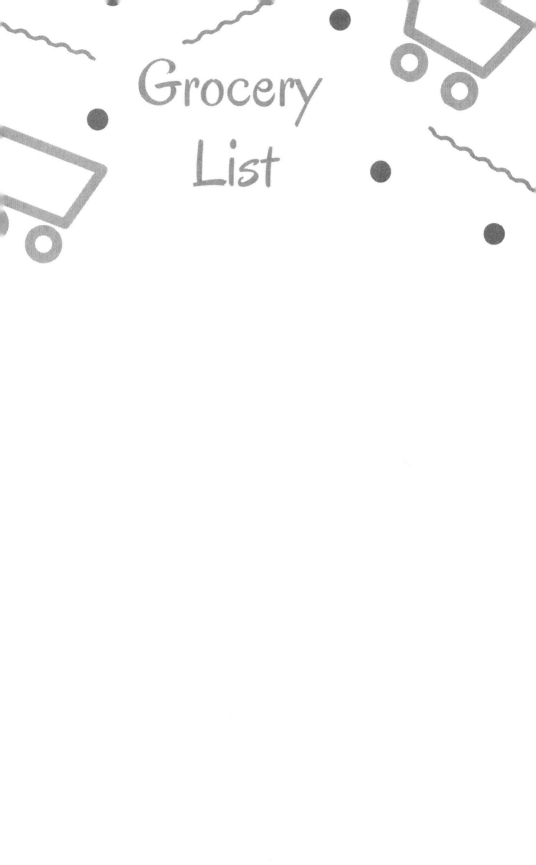

DATE:

YESTERDAY'S WIN:

TODAY'S GOAL:

I THING I'M GRATEFUL FOR:

TO DO'S:

EXERCISE:

BREAKFAST

LUNCH

DINNER

SNACKS

WATER

DATE:

YESTERDAY'S WIN:

TODAY'S GOAL:

I THING I'M GRATEFUL FOR:

TO DO'S:

EXERCISE:

BREAKFAST

LUNCH

DINNER

SNACKS

WATER

DATE:

YESTERDAY'S WIN:

TODAY'S GOAL:

I THING I'M GRATEFUL FOR:

TO DO'S:

EXERCISE:

BREAKFAST

LUNCH

DINNER

SNACKS

WATER

DATE:

YESTERDAY'S WIN:

TODAY'S GOAL:

I THING I'M GRATEFUL FOR:

TO DO'S:

EXERCISE:

BREAKFAST

LUNCH

DINNER

SNACKS

WATER

DATE:

YESTERDAY'S WIN:

TODAY'S GOAL:

I THING I'M GRATEFUL FOR:

TO DO'S:

EXERCISE:

BREAKFAST

LUNCH

DINNER

SNACKS

WATER

DATE:

YESTERDAY'S WIN:

TODAY'S GOAL:

I THING I'M GRATEFUL FOR:

TO DO'S:

EXERCISE:

BREAKFAST

LUNCH

DINNER

SNACKS

WATER

DATE:

YESTERDAY'S WIN:

BREAKFAST

TODAY'S GOAL:

LUNCH

1 THING I'M GRATEFUL FOR:

TO DO'S:

DINNER

EXERCISE:

SNACKS

WATER

Weekly Reflection

3 Wins This Week:

What Needs Improvement?

Actions Towards Improvement:

End Of Month Check In

Ending Weight: Ending BMI:

Non Scale Victories This Month :

Updated Measurements

Neck: Waist:

Bust: Thigh:

Hips: Arm:

How Do You Feel?

Month Goals

Starting Weight: Starting BMI:

4 WK WEIGHT LOSS GOAL: _____

Non Scale Goal:

Exercise Goal:

Action Plan:

Reward:

30 Day Habit Tracker

Habits To Grow: Habits To Cut:

Habit:

1 2 3 4 5 6 7 8 9 10 11 12 13 14 15 16 17
18 19 20 21 22 23 24 25 26 27 28 29 30

Habit:

1 2 3 4 5 6 7 8 9 10 11 12 13 14 15 16 17
18 19 20 21 22 23 24 25 26 27 28 29 30

Habit:

1 2 3 4 5 6 7 8 9 10 11 12 13 14 15 16 17
18 19 20 21 22 23 24 25 26 27 28 29 30

Habit:

1 2 3 4 5 6 7 8 9 10 11 12 13 14 15 16 17
18 19 20 21 22 23 24 25 26 27 28 29 30

NOTES

MONTH:

WEEK AT A GLANCE

WEIGHT: _____

EVENTS TO PLAN AROUND	MINI GOAL THIS WEEK
☐	
☐	
☐	**WORDS OF SELF ENCOURAGEMENT**
☐	
☐	

WEEK MEAL PLAN

	BKFST.	LUNCH	DINNER	SNACKS	CALS.
MON.					
TUE.					
WED.					
THUR.					

	BKFST.	LUNCH	DINNER	SNACKS	CALS.
FRI.					
SAT.					
SUN.					

SELF LOVE PROMPT:

TAKE SOME TIME THIS WEEK TO CREATE A SPACE JUST
FOR YOU. SOMEWHERE AT HOME WHERE YOU CAN SIT AND
BE STILL WITH YOUR THOUGHTS. CREATE YOUR OWN
LITTLE ZEN ZONE WITH CANDLES OR THINGS YOU ENJOY!
SPEND SOME TIME THERE FOR YOURSELF WEEKLY.

Grocery List

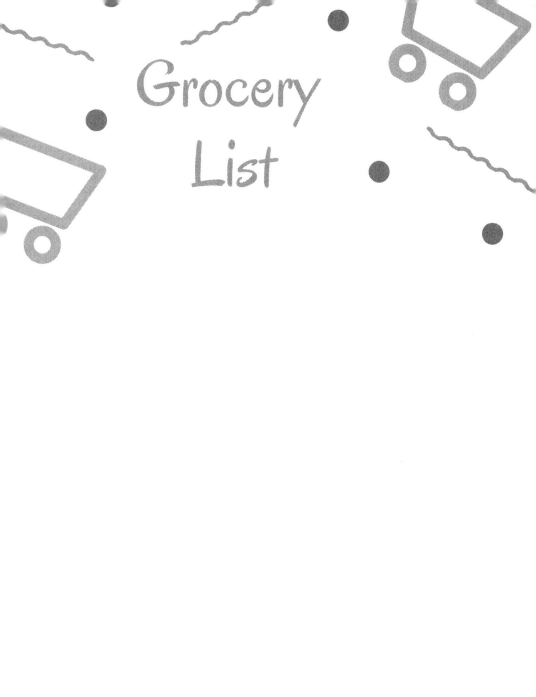

DATE:

YESTERDAY'S WIN:

TODAY'S GOAL:

I THING I'M GRATEFUL FOR:

TO DO'S:

EXERCISE:

BREAKFAST

LUNCH

DINNER

SNACKS

WATER

DATE:

YESTERDAY'S WIN:

TODAY'S GOAL:

I THING I'M GRATEFUL FOR:

TO DO'S:

EXERCISE:

BREAKFAST

LUNCH

DINNER

SNACKS

WATER

DATE:

YESTERDAY'S WIN:

TODAY'S GOAL:

I THING I'M GRATEFUL FOR:

TO DO'S:

EXERCISE:

BREAKFAST

LUNCH

DINNER

SNACKS

WATER

DATE:

YESTERDAY'S WIN:

TODAY'S GOAL:

1 THING I'M GRATEFUL FOR:

TO DO'S:

EXERCISE:

BREAKFAST

LUNCH

DINNER

SNACKS

WATER

DATE:

YESTERDAY'S WIN:

BREAKFAST

TODAY'S GOAL:

I THING I'M GRATEFUL FOR:

LUNCH

TO DO'S:

DINNER

EXERCISE:

SNACKS

WATER

DATE:

YESTERDAY'S WIN:

TODAY'S GOAL:

I THING I'M GRATEFUL FOR:

TO DO'S:

EXERCISE:

BREAKFAST

LUNCH

DINNER

SNACKS

WATER

DATE:

YESTERDAY'S WIN:

TODAY'S GOAL:

1 THING I'M GRATEFUL FOR:

TO DO'S:

EXERCISE:

BREAKFAST

LUNCH

DINNER

SNACKS

WATER

Weekly Reflection

3 Wins This Week:

What Needs Improvement?

Actions Towards Improvement:

WEEK AT A GLANCE

WEIGHT: _____

EVENTS TO PLAN AROUND	MINI GOAL THIS WEEK
☐	
☐	
☐	**WORDS OF SELF ENCOURAGEMENT**
☐	
☐	

WEEK MEAL PLAN

	BKFST.	LUNCH	DINNER	SNACKS	CALS.
MON.					
TUE.					
WED.					
THUR.					

	BKFST.	LUNCH	DINNER	SNACKS	CALS.
FRI.					
SAT.					
SUN.					

SELF LOVE PROMPT:

DESCRIBE YOURSELF THROUGH THE EYES OF A LOVED
ONE. TAKE THE TIME TO WRITE THIS DOWN IN A JOURNAL.
FEEL FREE TO ASK A LOVED ONE TO DESCRIBE YOU IF YOU
AREN'T SURE. VIEWING YOURSELF IN THE EYES OF
SOMEONE THAT LOVES YOU CAN ALTER YOUR
PERSPECTIVE AND CAUSE POSITIVE BELIEFS.

Grocery
List

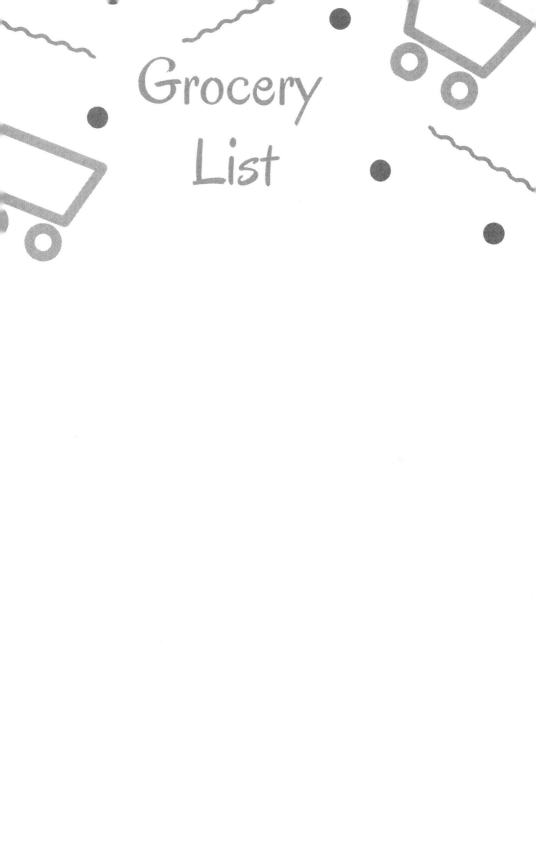

DATE:

YESTERDAY'S WIN:

TODAY'S GOAL:

1 THING I'M GRATEFUL FOR:

TO DO'S:

EXERCISE:

BREAKFAST

LUNCH

DINNER

SNACKS

WATER

DATE:

YESTERDAY'S WIN:

TODAY'S GOAL:

I THING I'M GRATEFUL FOR:

TO DO'S:

EXERCISE:

BREAKFAST

LUNCH

DINNER

SNACKS

WATER

DATE:

YESTERDAY'S WIN:

BREAKFAST

TODAY'S GOAL:

LUNCH

I THING I'M GRATEFUL FOR:

TO DO'S:

DINNER

EXERCISE:

SNACKS

WATER

DATE:

YESTERDAY'S WIN:

TODAY'S GOAL:

I THING I'M GRATEFUL FOR:

TO DO'S:

EXERCISE:

BREAKFAST

LUNCH

DINNER

SNACKS

WATER

DATE:

YESTERDAY'S WIN:

TODAY'S GOAL:

I THING I'M GRATEFUL FOR:

TO DO'S:

EXERCISE:

BREAKFAST

LUNCH

DINNER

SNACKS

WATER

DATE:

YESTERDAY'S WIN:

TODAY'S GOAL:

I THING I'M GRATEFUL FOR:

TO DO'S:

EXERCISE:

BREAKFAST

LUNCH

DINNER

SNACKS

WATER

DATE:

YESTERDAY'S WIN:

BREAKFAST

TODAY'S GOAL:

I THING I'M GRATEFUL FOR:

LUNCH

TO DO'S:

DINNER

EXERCISE:

SNACKS

WATER

Weekly Reflection

3 Wins This Week:

What Needs Improvement?

Actions Towards Improvement:

WEEK AT A GLANCE

WEIGHT: _____

EVENTS TO PLAN AROUND	MINI GOAL THIS WEEK
☐	
☐	
☐	**WORDS OF SELF ENCOURAGEMENT**
☐	
☐	

WEEK MEAL PLAN

	BKFST.	LUNCH	DINNER	SNACKS	CALS.
MON.					
TUE.					
WED.					
THUR.					

	BKFST.	LUNCH	DINNER	SNACKS	CALS.
FRI.					
SAT.					
SUN.					

SELF LOVE PROMPT:

AS YOU GO THROUGH YOUR WEEK WRITE DOWN 3 THINGS
A DAY THAT MADE YOU SMILE. BY THE END OF THE WEEK
YOU SHOULD HAVE 21 THINGS. HOW CAN YOU START
ADDING THESE THINGS INTO YOUR DAILY ROUTINE MORE.

Grocery
List

DATE:

YESTERDAY'S WIN:

TODAY'S GOAL:

I THING I'M GRATEFUL FOR:

TO DO'S:

EXERCISE:

BREAKFAST

LUNCH

DINNER

SNACKS

WATER

DATE:

YESTERDAY'S WIN:

TODAY'S GOAL:

I THING I'M GRATEFUL FOR:

TO DO'S:

EXERCISE:

BREAKFAST

LUNCH

DINNER

SNACKS

WATER

DATE:

YESTERDAY'S WIN:

TODAY'S GOAL:

I THING I'M GRATEFUL FOR:

TO DO'S:

EXERCISE:

BREAKFAST

LUNCH

DINNER

SNACKS

WATER

DATE:

YESTERDAY'S WIN:

TODAY'S GOAL:

I THING I'M GRATEFUL FOR:

TO DO'S:

EXERCISE:

BREAKFAST

LUNCH

DINNER

SNACKS

WATER

DATE:

YESTERDAY'S WIN:

TODAY'S GOAL:

I THING I'M GRATEFUL FOR:

TO DO'S:

EXERCISE:

BREAKFAST

LUNCH

DINNER

SNACKS

WATER

DATE:

YESTERDAY'S WIN:

BREAKFAST

TODAY'S GOAL:

I THING I'M GRATEFUL FOR:

LUNCH

TO DO'S:

DINNER

EXERCISE:

SNACKS

WATER

DATE:

YESTERDAY'S WIN:

TODAY'S GOAL:

I THING I'M GRATEFUL FOR:

TO DO'S:

EXERCISE:

BREAKFAST

LUNCH

DINNER

SNACKS

WATER

Weekly Reflection

3 Wins This Week:

What Needs Improvement?

Actions Towards Improvement:

WEEK AT A GLANCE

WEIGHT: _____

EVENTS TO PLAN AROUND	MINI GOAL THIS WEEK
☐	
☐	
☐	**WORDS OF SELF ENCOURAGEMENT**
☐	
☐	

WEEK MEAL PLAN

	BKFST.	LUNCH	DINNER	SNACKS	CALS.
MON.					
TUE.					
WED.					
THUR.					

	BKFST.	LUNCH	DINNER	SNACKS	CALS.
FRI.					
SAT.					
SUN.					

SELF LOVE PROMPT:

START YOUR MORNINGS WITH BREATHING. INHALE FOR 5
FULL SECONDS. HOLD YOUR BREATH FOR 5-FULL
SECONDS. EXHALE FOR 5-FULL SECONDS. REPEAT 3-5
TIMES. USE THROUGHOUT THE DAY WHEN FEELING
STRESSED.

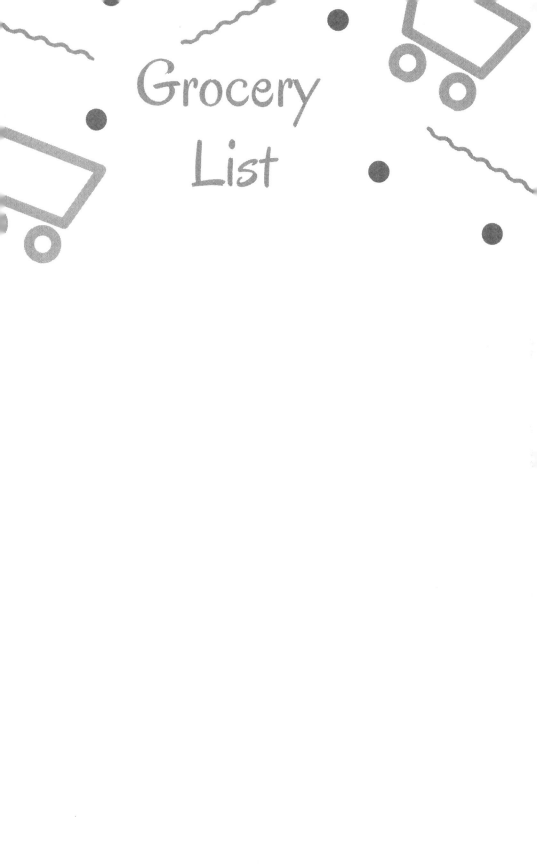

Grocery List

DATE:

YESTERDAY'S WIN:

TODAY'S GOAL:

I THING I'M GRATEFUL FOR:

TO DO'S:

EXERCISE:

BREAKFAST

LUNCH

DINNER

SNACKS

WATER

DATE:

YESTERDAY'S WIN:

TODAY'S GOAL:

I THING I'M GRATEFUL FOR:

TO DO'S:

EXERCISE:

BREAKFAST

LUNCH

DINNER

SNACKS

WATER

DATE:

YESTERDAY'S WIN:

BREAKFAST

TODAY'S GOAL:

LUNCH

I THING I'M GRATEFUL FOR:

TO DO'S:

DINNER

EXERCISE:

SNACKS

WATER

DATE:

YESTERDAY'S WIN:

TODAY'S GOAL:

I THING I'M GRATEFUL FOR:

TO DO'S:

EXERCISE:

BREAKFAST

LUNCH

DINNER

SNACKS

WATER

DATE:

YESTERDAY'S WIN:

TODAY'S GOAL:

I THING I'M GRATEFUL FOR:

TO DO'S:

EXERCISE:

BREAKFAST

LUNCH

DINNER

SNACKS

WATER

DATE:

YESTERDAY'S WIN:

TODAY'S GOAL:

I THING I'M GRATEFUL FOR:

TO DO'S:

EXERCISE:

BREAKFAST

LUNCH

DINNER

SNACKS

WATER

DATE:

YESTERDAY'S WIN:

TODAY'S GOAL:

I THING I'M GRATEFUL FOR:

TO DO'S:

EXERCISE:

BREAKFAST

LUNCH

DINNER

SNACKS

WATER

Weekly Reflection

3 Wins This Week:

What Needs Improvement?

Actions Towards Improvement:

End Of Month Check In

Ending Weight: Ending BMI:

Non Scale Victories This Month :

Updated Measurements

Neck: Waist:

Bust: Thigh:

Hips: Arm:

How Do You Feel?

Made in the USA
San Bernardino, CA
19 March 2019